BIPOLAR
Heaven and Hell

GEORGE "MANY WATERS" DAVIS

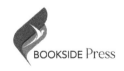
BOOKSIDE Press

Bipolar Heaven and Hell © 2022 George "Many Waters" Davis

ISBN:

Paperback	978-1-998784-36-3
Ebook	978-1-998784-37-0

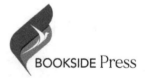

BOOKSIDE Press

BookSide Press
877-741-8091
www.booksidepress.com
orders@booksidepress.com

CONTENTS

DEDICATION

As I was writing this book, I was thinking of the many people down through the years that have helped me with my bipolar disorder. Some of these people have been those I have met when I was hospitalized.

However, most are my family members.

My wife, Barbara, has always tried to stick by me even when she didn't understand what was going on. My three children, Deborah, Stacie and Stephen have always tried to support me when they could. My daughters have done the computer work for me on this project. My mother has also been deeply affected by my disorder but has always been there for me.

I also want to thank my brother, Buddy and my two sisters, Sharon and Mary for continuing to support me.

I have been dealing with bipolar disorder for over 40 years now. It is not just a personal disorder; it is a family one too. Everyone near you is affected.

Last but not least, I want to thank the Lord Jesus Christ. Through His Holy Spirit, He has picked me up and encouraged me to keep on trying.

Thanks to all of you, even those I haven't mentioned.

INTRODUCTION

Bipolar Heaven and Hell is a result of over 40 years of dealing with this disorder. When you have dealt with it this long, you are able to see the symptoms and recognize them in others. It is my hope that this book reaches these people and helps them recognize the symptoms.

It is also my hope that families who have a member that is bipolar will read this book and have a better idea what their family member is dealing with.

People who have been dealing with bipolar disorder for quite some time will come to a place where they realize they can have a happy, healthy and productive life. Do not give up.

Psalms 139:14 I will praise thee for I am fearfully and wonderfully made.

CHAPTER I

Purpose

Greetings, if you are reading this little book, chances are you have a bipolar disorder or know someone who does. It may even be a family member. I am in my 60's now and had my first bipolar episode in 1972. I was in Vietnam in the infantry and had no idea what was transpiring at the time. Three years later I ended up in a mental institution and 3 years after that another mental institution. In 1978, I was diagnosed, by a German doctor, with bipolar disorder. At present, I have been dealing with this disorder for over 40 years. As you read this, please keep in mind, I am not a doctor.

This entire book is from a patient's point of view. I wish I had all the answers and a cure, but I don't! My purpose for writing this is many folds, but can be summed up into 4 or 5 basic reasons. During the course of my disorder, I have been in a mental hospital 12 times (and counting). My heart goes out to anyone with bipolar disorder and my hope is that this little book can help. I have also learned that bipolar is not just an individual disorder. It is a family disorder that affects not only close family members, although it usually affects them the most, it affects everyone the individual comes in contact with. It is my hope and purpose that this book helps these individuals have a better understanding of bipolar disorder.

Purpose is something we all need in our lives. Sometimes people with bipolar illness lose this vision. But now I believe that with proper medication and a good psychiatrist, bipolar individuals can live a happy functioning life.

I also believe that having a healthy spiritual foundation is very important. When we have Jesus and His God in our lives, it gives the bipolar individual a force within to talk to and reason things over with. Most of the people I know that have passed through the dark ages, so to speak, have some kind of spiritual foundation in their lives. This helps them function on a more even keel. As I end this chapter, it is my hope and prayer that all people with bipolar disorder can and will become happy, healthy functioning individuals.

As far as purpose is concerned, try to set small goals and do one at a time. Each time you finish one give yourself a little reward. You may not feel like you have a purpose. But you will find out that you have many. Help another person sometimes. This can help you build your own self esteem.

CHAPTER 2

Admit

This is perhaps the hardest step in the whole bipolar disorder process. No one wants to feel like there is something wrong with them. The truth of the matter is most human beings have something wrong with them, either physically or psychiatrically. The statement 'I'm perfect and you are not' is not the truth. Personally, I don't know anyone who is perfect. In fact, the word perfect is a relative word; Perfect relative to what? There is nothing, at all, to be ashamed of. People seek outside help for all kinds of things in their lives. If there is any shame at all, it may come at the end of your life and you look back and didn't seek help, when you could have been a happy individual making contributions to this life and this world. It is always the 'I' in us that has to make the change or choice. Life in the human flesh is not an easy task. However, there is so much we can learn in our short time here. Let's face it, in view of eternity, 100 years is a short time. Don't get trapped in the blame game. Blaming something or someone else never made a decision for anyone. It is always and ever will be the 'I' in you that makes the change and choice. Listen to all people's opinions but ultimately let the 'I' in you be the one that makes the choice.

Now, this book is mainly for individuals that have been diagnosed with bipolar disorder, their family members and people they come into contact with. But dealing with bipolar for over 40 years, I can't help but mention the people I have come in contact with that I believed to have some of the symptoms. Usually, they are using some form of self-medication. To get them to admit they need help and seek it is extremely hard. Talk to them about your own bipolar disorder or someone you know that has the disorder.

Suggest this may be a possibility but there is help available. You may be able to talk to one of their loved ones but this is about all you can do. It is sad sometimes, until someone is willing to admit they need help and take the next step (seek it) your hands are tied. Pray for them, God can bring about change.

This also applies to someone that has been diagnosed bipolar but is running away from the problem. If there is a second step to admit, it has to be sought help. They may be willing to admit 'yes, I have a bipolar disorder' but are unwilling to take the medication that has been prescribed. For this reason or that, there are 101 bad reasons not to take medication. It is important to take your medicine on a regular basis. The single extremely important thing is to stay on your medication. When you are manic, you feel like you don't need medication. If you stop taking it you are going to get in trouble. Unfortunately, bipolar disorder requires medication. There is no shame or failure in that. It's not your fault. The sooner you accept this the better off you will be. I can't emphasize this enough. I played this game for years, only to end up in a mental institution or jail once again. Be open and honest with yourself and your doctors. Be willing to explore. There are so many good medications out there now, in 2018, for bipolar disorder you wouldn't believe it and they are always coming up with newer and better ones. You may want to try this when you are willing to seek help again, mark your calendar and try the medication your doctor prescribes for two weeks (three would be better). Believe me, if I can do it you can too. Look at it this way, you have only disharmony to lose and peace and tranquility to gain. It's not unusual to go through 1 or 2 medications that don't work. But don't give up. I believe in this age there is the right one for you out there. Don't be dismayed. What I am suggesting will take sacrifice and change. But the end results are well worth the effort.

Accept yourself just as you are, baggage and all. God accepts you that way. God doesn't look so much at us as what we are at this moment, but what we can become. It is a good place to start, right where you are. Remember I said the 'I' in you is the only thing that can bring about change. Change takes place in the moment. The moment the 'I' in you sets the course, change begins. The journey never ends, in this life or the next. We always and forever will keep growing and learning. God creates us that way, in God's likeness.

Ok, so we have a bipolar disorder. What are we going to do about it? Keep moving forward not backward. People have all kinds of disorders in the human body; cancer, diabetes, etc. It's by far not the worst disorder you could have. In fact, in my 60's, I can now look back and say dealing with bipolar disorder has taught me more about life than many other experiences.

You have heard we can only live one day at a time. This is truth. But it goes even deeper than that. All changes take place in what I call the 'Isma' dimension, or the eternal now. Take the heartbeat for example. In three heartbeats the future becomes the present and the present becomes the past. It is the eternal now I am speaking of. It's a breakdown in time from one day to the eternal moment. All change takes place in the moment or 'Isma' dimension. What is...is. We can't change that. We can only deal with the circumstances at hand. A wise man once said 'One of the most powerful things human beings possess is thought and the power to manifest it'. A day can be long, the eternal moment is easier to deal with. Sit down in your soul in a state of rest as much as possible now. Learn to try your thoughts, whether they be positive or negative, good or evil. Live in the moment.

You will find out that most people with bipolar disorder are very creative in one area or another. If you have been bipolar for some time and are seeking help or counsel, you have probably heard the term 'grandiose idea'. When I first heard that term it had a negative connotation. Like man, you are bipolar and have grandiose ideas. All thoughts can get you in trouble sometimes without counsel. I have learned there is a positive side to them also. Sometimes a grandiose idea can be a good one.

I have learned that seeking counsel is always a good thing. Wise people all down through the ages have done this. For me, my first counsel is with my wife of 40 plus years. From there I seek out people that may have the most knowledge about the subject at hand. So just because you may have been deemed as having grandiose ideas, don't disregard all of them. You may disregard a good one. So, in closing to this chapter, admit you need help and seek it out. There's a very good chance you will find it. Don't be ashamed you have a bipolar disorder. People that are not going through it, do not understand. That's ok. There are many things we can't understand unless we experience it ourselves. So, keep moving in a forward direction. It can and will get better.

CHAPTER 3

Cycles and Circles

Greetings. When I conceived the idea to write this book, I didn't want to make it a religious book, so to speak. However, Jesus lives in my heart and is as much a part of my day as anyone or anything else. I am a Christian and feel honored to be so. You have heard me use words like God, pray and Christ. You will hear them again because much of my learning has come from my spirituality.

Now what I'm about to write about may not apply to all people with bipolar disorder, but it seems to be this way with me and many others. Have you ever heard or read about the alpha and omega sacred circle of knowledge? It is a circle much like a halo. When you begin on the circle to learn about this or that you begin a journey around the circle. The end of the cycle is where you begin and it starts all over again. The sacred circle of learning and knowledge never ends. I have come to look at bipolar disorder like a circle or cycle. Take for example the clock, put mania at 12:00 and depression at 6:00. It seems what goes up must come down. Let's say we start in a state of mania at 12:00. The clock moves at different rates of speed, at different times for certain individuals. A manic episode could last for several months, but the clock is turning and 6:00 or a state of depression, usually follows most of the time.

The more severe the manic episode, the more severe the depression episode. This is where medication is so important. There is no cure for bipolar disorder, that I know of, but there are lots of good medications to help with mania and depression. The medications keep both from being so severe. So, stay in close contact with your doctors during both states, mania and depression. If there is any way possible, try and get in a bipolar group. I joined one a few years ago and it has helped me a lot. It gives you a chance to be around other people who are experiencing or have experienced most of the things you are going through. Again, no two souls are the same. It is very hard for someone that is not bipolar to understand the thought process of someone that is. In my group, there is a doctor and a psychiatrist. They can discuss medications and prescribe something different if you need to change. There are different medications sometimes for the mania state and the depression state. I will talk about that some time in a later chapter.

There is a world of difference between having a manic episode and going through a depression episode. Another thing that can help is getting off alone somewhere. Take a day trip alone to the mountains or the beach if you can. Try taking a nice long walk in the woods. There are many ways you can do it but getting off alone can help. Look back on your past experiences with bipolar and see if you can see a pattern. If you do, it can help when dealing with this disorder. In my opinion, the depressions are the hardest part. However, if you see your bipolar disorder moving in a circle or cycle, it will pass. You will then move towards more enlightened states of mind. Most bipolar patients like the manic state better. It can reach almost 'heavenly' states at times, just as the depression can reach almost 'hellish' states. Balance and seeking counsel are the "keys". With the proper help, we can reach a balance so that the lows are not so low and the highs are not so high that they get you in deep trouble.

Over the years I have seen so many divorces because of bi-polar disorder, I pray this doesn't happen as much in the future. If you started your marriage off in a good loving relationship, chances are you still love and need each other. There are lots of reasons to get a divorce. There may be children involved. Ask yourself if not seeking help or taking medication is worth the pain of divorce. Over a period of years there have been times when I stopped seeing my doctors and quit taking my medications. Yes, I have heard my wife say "I can't deal with this anymore, I'm leaving". We have separated twice. But by the grace of God, I went back to taking my medications once again. When your spouse or family member sees you trying, it puts a whole different light on the subject. So be encouraged and don't give up. There is lots of help available, if we seek it. Study the patterns of your disorder, it helps.

CHAPTER 4

Symptoms

Greetings. It seemed important to write about symptoms. How long have you been bipolar? This is an important question to ask as we begin this chapter. Again, this book is mainly for those people who have been diagnosed bipolar but could help with people you come in contact with who may be bipolar and haven't been diagnosed. I have had this happen several times. It may be a little easier for me to pick them out since I have experienced it for so many years. This chapter on symptoms may help with that.

In the sixties, bipolar was called manic depression. Jimi Hendrix wrote a song about it. So I'm going to start this with the manic side of bipolar. Most bipolar patients love the manic side it's almost intoxicating. This is the 'feel good' time for most. For me, this is when I feel great. You're enthusiastic, you have a lot of energy, usually you require less sleep than most. Once it starts, it progresses. As it progresses, your thoughts become more and more excessive. This is called "racing thoughts". After a while it starts interfering with your sleep, you find yourself needing less and less. These are states of mania. I have gone for weeks on 3-4 hours of sleep at night and sometimes I have even gone days with no sleep at all. When you are in this state of mind, most of your senses are heightened. This is where we usually have our 'heavenly' or 'divine' experiences, even grandiose ideas. Usually this leads to some kind of breakdown. Mania can become very irrational and dangerous to yourself and others. You can reach a point where you have lost control and need intervention. Our emotions start to be more and more elevated. Some develop issues with anger. First, we must realize that most anger comes from past hurt. So, keep that in mind if you are dealing with an anger issue. Talking excessively can also be a sign. People who are manic usually have so much to say that most of the time they dominate the conversation. Rapid mood swings can sometimes occur. This is called 'rapid cycling'.

If you have been diagnosed with bipolar disorder and are taking your medication, it is time for a change or something in addition to what you are already taking. Most likely a new medication to replace what you are on or adjusting your dose can help a lot. I don't need to say what to do if you are not taking your medication. Call your doctor first. Medication takes time to get into or back into your system. Tell your doctor your symptoms. There may be something new they can suggest at the time. There are many expressions of mania, each person is different. These are only a few suggestions to help out.

Now I'm going to discuss the depression side of bipolar disorder. A doctor once told me that it is the hardest part of the disorder. All humans function on highs and lows. This is normal. When you are clinically diagnosed, your brain is not functioning properly and the highs and lows get extreme and out of control. This is where medication is needed. Depression usually doesn't happen overnight. It is a process just like the mania side. However, in states of mania we don't want to change because it feels almost divine at times. It's not easy, in fact, being bipolar may be one of the most challenging things you ever have to deal with. It's not the worst, but is difficult. Once we realize we are going through deeper states of depression, it is a little easier to seek help. The depth of the depression may vary from individual to individual. A deep state of depression is hell on earth. Again, like mania, your emotions are intensified. You may feel tired all the time and start sleeping more than usual. Little things seem monumental, to a point that it almost drives you crazy. It comes if you don't seek help. Suicidal thoughts can occur during deep states of depression. In fact, most people that commit suicide are going through deep depression. Do you hear voices? This is also a sign in both mania and depression as well as in other mental disorders. If you do hear voices, don't listen to them when it comes to suicide. It is never a salvation. I tried once back in 1982, I won't go into detail but God delivered me from it. It scared me so badly that I promised Him I would never again attempt to take my life. I wish I could tell you I have bipolar disorder down pat but I can't, because I don't.

It is a day to day, moment to moment struggle. However, it gets better if we don't give up and get the right help. I don't want to sound like a pill pusher because I'm not. I don't like taking medication any more than necessary. Deep states of depression can bring you to a halt. There are additional medications that can help bring you out of it. So, remember the bipolar clock is still ticking around and this too will pass. If you persevere and seek the right help, you will move on to more enlightened states of mind.

It is all about balance. The objective is to not go too high or too low. Personally, I don't know how to achieve that balance without the proper medications and above all God in your life. I can honestly say without the living Christ in my life, I would not be here in this present moment. The heavenly counsel that He can offer in your heart and mind can make all the difference in the world, whether you are dealing with bipolar or just plain life itself.

Life in the human flesh is not an easy task. Someone once told me life is a continual process of solving one problem after the other. Problems never stop popping up, but it is the attitude we approach them with that is most important. We can always look around us and say this one or that one has it made however, all human souls must face tribulations of some kind.

Long periods of sadness may be a sign of depression. Some other signs are really low energy levels, being tired all of the time, getting panic attacks, feeling like you are going to die, irritability, getting upset over little things you normally wouldn't pay much attention to. Here again there are many symptoms of depression. If these symptoms continue for a long period of time, two weeks or more, or you begin to have suicidal thoughts, call your doctor right away. Suicidal thoughts are nothing to play around with. If this happens, your depression is going from bad to worse. Again, I say, get help. If you have been bipolar for quite some time, the depression usually passes and you move on to a better state of mind.

The more experienced you are with bipolar the more you are able to recognize the triggers that begin to set off mania or depression. If we pay attention to these triggers, maybe they can help us from going too high or too low. Take note of your triggers, they vary for each individual. Stress plays a part in every individual's mental health. Two or three heavy stresses can be a trigger, it is for me. But stress also is one of those things in life that doesn't go away. Here again, it's how we deal with stress in our mind that counts.

Pray to be a teachable spirit. God loves a teachable soul and can move us to heights we have never known through the lessons we learned. Explore and try new ways to deal with things. If one thing is not working, try something else. The hardest part is to just keep moving in a forward motion in your mind. We tend to get stuck sometimes in one frame of mind or another. This is normal. If we practice being a teachable spirit, it won't last but for so long. New ideas and new things to try have a way of coming up.

You are an awesome creature. I read a book one time called "Fearfully and Wonderfully Made" by Dr. Paul Brand. He is a missionary and this orthopedic surgeon worked in India treating and caring for people with leprosy for over 20 years. Dr. Brand wrote about how fearfully and wonderfully made the human body truly is. In God's eyes, you are a spirit with a soul. So believed Dr. Paul Brand. The heights and depths of spirit and soul has not been told by man. I am the spirit of Butch and you are the spirit of you. This is your vibration or aura. We usually all agree that different people put off different vibrations or "vibes". Your spirit touches every living cell in your body. It is the sustainer of life. This is why when your spirit comes out of your body, the body ceases to function. The spirit moves on to a new dimension. All spirits are being prepared for eternity but we are not all going to the same place. This is why Jesus taught love your neighbor as yourself. Red, yellow, black or white we are all one.

You can't harm someone else and not harm yourself. Likewise, you can't help someone and not help yourself on some level. We are that interconnected. Bear with me on some of this stuff. You are of great worth and need to know it.

You probably have heard that we are three-part beings, body, soul and spirit. This is true as God is also a three-part being and works basically on three planes or dimensions. A third part of you is spirit. The body changes from dimension to dimension. The human experience is only one level on the spiritual path of life. You are more than body and spirit; you have a soul. This, too, is a great mystery as many things in life are but it's the great mysteries in life that keep us seeking to learn and grow. I believe that soul is the entirety of our essence and you will probably hear me say this again and again. Jesus taught 'what does it profit a man if he gains the whole world but loses his own soul?' Like I said, you are of great worth though you might not feel that way at any given moment. Do you like yourself? Some may say yes but not all. Some people just plain say 'I don't like myself'. I have felt this way many times, mostly when in states of depression.

Words are very powerful things but thoughts often manifest themselves into words also. We all know how the spoken word affects people around us. Thoughts affect the soul in much the same way. They can build or destroy. This is leading up to the next chapter which I will call "voices". First, I have to mention some basic foundations in order to approach that subject. To sum up this chapter, there are many signs and symptoms that lead us up to states of mania and depression. There is a Japanese word I learned some years ago, Kaizen, which has to do with achievement but basically means 'constant, never-ending improvement'. So, keep on trying different ways to improve your bipolar disorder.

There are also other ways to help, along with medications. Proper vitamins and minerals along with a little exercise can help a lot. This is an area I am starting to work on now. My doctor suggested it in addition to lithium which is the medication I'm taking right now. It may not work for you but it is working well for me at present. So, explore, try new ways to deal with your bipolar disorder. Study your triggers, try and catch the symptoms of mania and depression before they get you in trouble.

CHAPTER 5

Voices

In the last chapter, you heard me ask the question 'do you hear voices'? Although hearing voices is one of the symptoms of bipolar disorder, it deserves a chapter of its own. It is still a gray area with doctors and psychiatrists. Most say 'Well, it's all in your mind'. This may be partly true but not completely.

We all agree the human body is an awesome creation. Have you ever heard of the 7 chakras of the body? It is an eastern teaching having to do with energy centers in our body in which energy flows. It starts at your feet and comes up to your head. There are two 'chakras' that I would like to talk about, heart space and mind space. They are two different dimensions but they all affect us emotionally. You have heard people say 'my heart tells me this or that'. Well, there is more to that than most are aware of. Heart space is the very core of intent. From there it goes to your mind, to be reasoned over and then your body is able to manifest it into the world, be it good or evil, positive or negative, right or wrong. God is creating all human beings with reasoning at the moment. Creation is an eternal motion, at the same time creation is continually being born and dissolved.

In the last chapter we talked about the power of the spoken word. In truth, words are spirit. You can't see them but they are a powerful force that can build or destroy. Basically, human beings have two tongues or two ways to speak. We all know our flesh tongue or vocal cords which is how we talk and express ourselves. This is important to note, we must be living active human beings to do this and have this power. If someone or something foul convinces us to commit suicide, we lose this power of human expression in this dimension. There is a victory on one level for evil, when this happens. Your second tongue, or voice chords, is in your mind. This is the voice we talk to ourselves with. I call it the spirit tongue. This is the voice of our consciousness that moves on when your spirit comes out of your body upon death of the flesh. So, we see how powerful words are. Thoughts also manifest themselves as words at times. However, they also have a powerful effect on the soul's state of being. This may seem a little confusing at first but as time goes on you will understand it more.

There is another avenue where voices or words can come from. Have you ever been doing something, maybe driving down the road alone, and a voice spoke to you but there was something different this time? The voice seemed to be coming from somewhere other than yourself. It happens to some people more than others. If you talk to people about it, some but not all, will have had this experience. Do you believe in guardian angels? I do. Jesus taught, where children were concerned, 'woe unto them that harm the least of these little ones, for their angels are before God'. I believe that the human mind can be influenced by outside forces, both good and evil. You may not believe in demon possession. I didn't either until I was in a couple of state mental institutions because of my bipolar disorder. Some of the ungodly things I saw convinced me. So, you are bipolar and you hear voices. Its ok, many bipolar patients do. Don't be afraid or ashamed to talk about it. The old saying 'man up or woman up' and keep your problems to yourself, is just plain not good teaching.

The more you learn to express yourself, the healthier you become. I don't mean dump all your problems on everyone all the time. There is a right time and right people to do this with. Learn to judge your thoughts. The scale of positive and negative is a good place to start. It could be that God or your guardian angel gives you a couple words of encouragement. Accept this, you probably needed it at that moment. God and your guardian angel are one, so to speak. They are for you 100%, at all times. Good and evil is a little harsher scale to use but it is the truth. Some voices are just plain evil and lead to discontent and destruction. Like suicide for example. It's never, never God's will for you to kill yourself. These are the voices of negativity or evil. When you are having these kinds of thoughts, dispel them as soon as possible. Move your mind on to thinking about things good and positive.

It takes effort but if we keep trying to improve, the rewards can be great. You can be a happy, healthy bipolar individual with a good relationship and a healthy family structure. I'm working on it and I've seen it happen. I'm more on an even keel now than I have been for a long time. Do I have all the answers? Do I have bipolar down pat? No. I work on it day by day. You can do the same. Do you hear voices? You are not alone. You are among many. There is a good chance angel are in the midst. Jesus also taught beware, for you entertain angels in unawares. God works a lot of times through holy angels. This may not be the norm but I have communed with my guardian angel since I was 6 years old, from time to time. I believe there are angels all around us all of the time. This applies to all human beings. They are not usually visible to the human eye for some reason. This is called the universal law of faith. We as human beings are challenged to believe, by faith, in a universal creator we cannot see. It's by faith we begin to have a relationship with God. Christianity should be called relationship. It's much more about relationships than religion. Jesus' whole life from the time he was born until he rose from the grave was to enhance relationships with God and one another.

There is another universal law. Some people call it the 11th commandment. The law of love. Love is a spirit also. We can't see it but we all know it and the good effects it can have. The law of love pretty much sums up the Ten Commandments. If we love our neighbors, we won't steal from them, lie to them or seek to kill them. Holy angels must also follow universal laws. Some we know and many we don't yet. Angels are peculiar creatures. The word angel comes from the word messenger. Angels have little to do with form or appearance. There are many sects of angels in creation. In the hierarchy, there are seraphim and cherubim but all the holy angels are messengers of God. Three angels appeared to Abraham in the form of men and ate a meal with him. Jesus also appeared to his disciples after he rose from the dead and had meals with them. Not counting dreams, which is a whole different subject altogether, I have only seen an angel once. I was cutting grass one day on a riding mower, I was in a rather gleeful spirit. I was enjoying the sky and nature all around me. All of a sudden out of the corner of my eye I saw a man standing by the entrance to my drive way. The moment I focused on him; he streaked off into the sky. It only lasted a few seconds. It was a man in human form, no wings. Was it my guardian? I now believe it was. On some level, I believe that men deal with men and women deal with women. I was asking the question 'do men have male guardians and female have female ones?' I don't know at present but there is a good chance this could be true.

The mind is one of the most mysterious parts of the human body. If you are bipolar, your brain is firing off a little different than most. This is why bipolar disorder is a chemical imbalance. Admit you need help and seek it. Admitting alone is not enough. You must take the next step and seek help. You will feel better and the people around you will be proud of you for trying to do so. The main purpose of writing this book is, I pray, to help people with bipolar disorder. Again, I say it's only the 'I' in you that can do that. No one can do it for you, not even God. If you're seeking help, you will get assistance but only you can make the free will choice.

Here again, there are people that have been diagnosed with bipolar, accept it and seek help but are still struggling. Keep seeking help. There are new medications coming out all the time. There is a good chance there is the right one for you. If you're not in a bipolar group, find one if possible. I have a monthly meeting I attend. It has helped me a lot. If you hear a voice, in your mind and recognize it as being someone other than yourself, there is a good chance God and the holy angels are in the midst. The voices can be good or bad. There are other forces involved also, we all know. The voice that comes from good and the spirit of love is always positive. It is usually a still small voice in your mind. It builds, encourages and edifies you in a time of need, it's always there for you 101% of the time. With practice, you can learn to recognize these influences and use them to help you in your life. You may have a physical visitation while you are awake or while dreaming. God gets messages to us in our dream world. He did with people all through the bible. Most dreams are just dreams and part of the human experience. You may even remember them but every once in a while, we have one that stands out. Pay attention to your dreams, there may be some help in that avenue also. We as human beings are so interconnected with each other and the universe.

I felt it necessary to write a chapter on angels and voices. If you are bipolar and don't hear voices, that is ok too. No two souls are alike. You probably have plenty of other things to deal with at present. If you do hear voices in your mind, calling your name one day, don't be dismayed. Ask it 'who are you?' and wait for a reply. You may be surprised.

CHAPTER 6

Making Amends

S ometimes in the bipolar process, there is healing that needs to take place. Making financial mistakes usually work themselves out but making mistakes with other human beings does not always. We mentioned bipolar disorder is a family disorder as much as it is a personal one. Sometimes family members and friends get hurt. Using bipolar disorder as an excuse is not good just as an alcoholic uses drinking. No healing for anyone can take place.

I am writing this chapter because of my past experiences and believe me; I've made plenty of mistakes. Most were while on the manic cycle of the disorder. I pray you haven't done this but this chapter is for those that have. Making amends can change the present state of mind of those you have harmed as well as your own. Sometimes we have things hidden deep in our souls that affect us and we are not even aware of it. It takes a lot of courage to face your mistakes. It's not easy to be honest with yourself at times. The mind is great at playing cover up games. Never be afraid to ask for forgiveness from someone you may have harmed. The healing that can take place may surprise you. Most often these kinds of things transpire within the family because they are the ones closest to you. If you have some amends that need to be made, I would pray about it first for a while. You may want to make sort of a priority list in your mind or on paper, if necessary. There are usually one or two that need to be handled first. You may not be able to make amends with everyone. You may have moved and someone is no longer in your life, maybe a phone call can be made. Admitting you made a mistake and asking for forgiveness is the process you want to use. I have had to do this a few times but I've never run across anyone that wasn't willing to forgive and put it behind them. It could be your spouse is the first person you need to talk to. It was in my case. Marriage doesn't have to end because of bipolar disorder. They can be healed.

I learned this process in a NA group but it works with bipolar disorder as well as with life in general. So, making amends, when possible, can free your spirit as well as the spirit of the individual involved. Getting these things out in the open can be healing for everyone. Any healing that takes place makes one a happier, healthier individual. You are better equipped to deal with things at hand in the present. If you do need to make amends, there is no time limit on it. Sometimes we need to use discretion. Choosing the right time and place can be just as important. My best results have been one on one or face to face. There may be a few tears that need to be shed, that's ok. We were told, in my generation, real men don't cry. So, we practiced keeping it all in. This is just plain not a good philosophy. Tear ducts are holy, God put them there for a very good reason. Sometimes a good cry is good for you, it can be a release. So don't be ashamed to shed a tear or two, it's healthy. I'll end this chapter with this, make amends when possible and use discretion and prayer.

CHAPTER 7
Self-Identity

Greetings, in this year, 2018. For the most part, this book has laid around idle on a shelf. I met a lady a few weeks ago that had written and published a book. She gave me her publisher's number and encouraged me to complete my book, this little book. It has been three years now since I wrote the last chapter and I feel like I have learned a lot more about bipolar disorder in that time span. Self-identity is all about how you feel about yourself. There is also what is called a dual diagnosis, for example, bipolar and P.T.S.D. or bipolar and schizophrenia. The majority of the world seems to have to put a label on everything. However, these labels can greatly affect how we feel about ourselves. In my 40 plus years of dealing with this bipolar, I have seen many people in mental hospitals lose their vision of hope and purpose. I have seen some and yes, even myself, feel as though they are worthless with not enough reason to keep on going. This usually takes place when they are going through days of depression. It is in this state most suicides occur. It literally gets so bad that you are ready to die and go on to the next life rather than bear the pain. If you feel like this, please seek help as soon as possible. This indeed is the negative side of bipolar disorder. Don't blame yourself for the way you feel. That is what most people do in this state of mind. Your brain simply is not producing the proper things it needs to function normally. Talk to a doctor and see a psychiatrist. Get your feelings out. Don't bottle them up inside. Life is a sacred journey. We are all indigenous to where we are born, no matter where that might be on earth. However, where you were born and the family you were raised in, has much to do with how you think and feel. Your personal journey from your cradle to the very present moment is how you feel and what state of mind you are in at present. Just for reference, we will call the very present moment 'Isma dimension'. It is always the 'present' or 'now moment'.

Man knows less about the human mind than any other organ in the body. It has been said that Einstein used only 10 percent of his brain and he is what we call a genius today. Wow, that leaves a lot to explore.

In one chapter in this book, I talked about grandiose ideas. They say when people with bipolar disorder are experiencing mania, they have a lot of grandiose ideas. That is not all together bad. As long as your idea comes to the sum of good, it is a good thing. People down through the ages, with grandiose ideas, have formed our history.

I have so many wounds on my heart because of what people have said or done to me because of my bipolar disorder. It is a lie from the devil. Remember the old saying we learned when we were young, 'sticks and stones will break my bones but words will never hurt me'? That is simply not true. Bones can be mended, but harsh or unkind words can wound a soul for a lifetime. Self-identity is very important to all of us, but it is of utmost importance to people that are labeled with a mental disorder. Often times bipolars even lose their identity. Whether this book makes it or not, is not as important to me now as it was three years age. I need to express myself and be myself.

You are loved much more than you know by our 'Creator'. You are a soul and a little 'spirit', a great thing.

Bill, a friend of mine, once told me 'you can't be anywhere except where you are' and it's absolutely true. Accept where you are right now. I have come to this realization often and I just plain did not like where I was. However, God gave us this beautiful little word: *Hope*. Everyone is different, God made us that way. No two snowflakes are the same. For me, it often helps to take a little time set apart from everyone and everything, just get off by myself. Take a drive down to the ocean, drive up to a mountain and park, or take a walk in the woods. Do whatever works for you.

Bipolar is something you will probably be dealing with the rest of your life, unless someone comes up with a cure. I still struggle with this myself. As I said earlier, there are a lot better medications available now than there were in 1975 when I was put into my first mental hospital. To me, the deep depression state is hell on earth and the hardest part of the disorder. They have a lot of anti-depressants and natural nutrients to help these days. Don't overlook the natural nutrients. Our bodies are a lot like the soil of the earth. It needs the proper minerals and nutrients to function properly and produce good crops. I felt it was important to write about self-identity. We are all different and no one is perfect. Sometimes people look down on people with mental disorders. It will affect how you feel about yourself, if you let it. Like I said before, words are spirit, they are like the wind, you can't see it but it's a powerful thing. I believe I talked about the great spiritual war that is going on between good and evil right now, in this dimension. I was learning under a wise native American elder a concept regarding our thinking process. It sounds kind of funny but there is a lot of truth in it. He said don't spell mind with a 'd', spell it with an 'e' on the end…'mine'. Like a mine field in a war zone. Yes, thoughts are powerful things. The Holy Scriptures also teaches us to 'try our thoughts and judge our thoughts'. Make a little mental note of this, it will help you.

Now, I have touched a bit on self-identity. It is such a universal concept. People have written hundreds of books about it, but I have tried to apply it to those that suffer with mental disorder. In the next chapter, I want to talk a bit about self-medicating.

CHAPTER 8

Self-Medicating

My eldest daughter suggested that I write a chapter on this topic. I am in my 60's now. As stated in chapter one, I had my first manic episode in 1972 when I was in Vietnam. At the time I had no idea what was happening to me. I knew something strange was going on but being in a war zone can do strange things to you. I came home in '72, got married in '74 to my beloved wife, Barbara, Little Wings. Between 1975 and 1978, I was hospitalized three times. In 1978, a German doctor diagnosed me with bipolar disorder. I was given lithium for the first time.

When you are in the military, most drink alcohol in their spare time and some smoke marijuana or do other drugs as well. When I came back from Vietnam, I was drinking and smoking marijuana. I pretty much stayed away from any chemical drugs; they scared me. I was a tug boat captain when I got drafted, so the company I worked for gave me my job back with all the raises included. Back in '72 a captain on a tug boat made pretty good money, so I had plenty to party with. I was 21 and I liked the ladies so that was the thing to do, party and try to pick up a woman. When I was diagnosed bipolar in '78, the first thing the doctors tell you is not to drink or do any drugs while taking the medication. They call it 'self-medicating'.

All human beings are creatures of habit, and they say old habits are hard to break and it is true. I did a little better for a while, but then I started moving into another manic episode. If you have never experienced a manic episode, it's hard to explain. The closest I can come is to say it feels like you are having a divine experience. Mania feels better than any drink or drug. You become so joyous and energized you are unable to sit still or sleep much.

This is an early warning. If you are drinking or doing drugs on top of this, you are about to get into *big* trouble. This is usually when people that are new to bipolar often stop taking their medications. I know because I have done it for years and have had to go into mental institutions on an average of every year to year and a half. You can self-medicate on either the depression or manic side. If you are doing it in excess, you are heading for a disaster.

A manic state could last weeks, months or even longer. You are entering into dimensions in your brain that the average human being doesn't experience. This is not altogether a bad thing but if you stop taking your medication it gets out of balance. You start having a hard time communicating with people. You may mess up your finances and can go into debt. Sometimes you think you are the only one right but the world is all wrong. There may be times when you don't seek help and your family has to green warrant you into the hospital. That means the law comes and picks you up and takes you for observation. If this happens, don't resist, because if you do, you will suffer the consequences. So, it's best to just go along.

How long have you been dealing with mental illness? This is an important question. As I said from the beginning, this book is from the patient's point of view. I am not a doctor and I don't have a cure. However, doctors have learned so much more about mental illness in this generation. It takes years sometimes to get bad habits in hand. Please stay on your medication. If that is not working, see your doctor and try something else.

Self-medicating covers many things. Medication is basically given to you for what ails you or to make you feel better. Everyone wants to feel better. There is nothing wrong with that. Self-medication also comes in many forms like alcohol as well as many kinds of drugs. Prescription drugs are a big problem right now. However, over eating, over spending and even sex can also be a form of self-medicating. It all comes down to use and abuse for most people. If you are bipolar or have another kind of mental illness, this may interfere with the diagnosis process or the medication given. If you are drinking or doing drugs every day, you may be self-medicating. If you are, and not taking your meds, you are going to crash and burn. That's one of the reasons I wrote about self-medication. So, use your head about it and be careful about self-medication. Do you have Christ Jesus in your life? Invite Him in now. This will be the most important thing you do in your life. This will give you ways and things you have never know about to help you overcome adversities.

Divine balance is what we all are looking for, humans with mental illness and those that don't have to deal with it. Be honest first with yourself and then all others. Arise and face your problems with prayer. You can do it. A wise man once said 'life is a series of dealing with one problem after another. They never stop. It's the way you deal with them that counts. So be careful with self-medicating and don't give up.

CHAPTER 9

Perspective

Greetings my people, welcome to eternity. Be at peace, my beloved, with any kind of mental disorder. You have suffered more than most. It's ok to ask any question, there are no bad ones, like why do I have to deal with the kind of things that go with mental illness? Sometimes it feels like you are an island in the stream and you are all alone. I understand completely but believe me, you have never been alone. It is all about perspective. What is your perspective at present? Eternity is a moving thing; it is always on the move. We change, sometimes daily, as we experience the gift of life. So be encouraged, we can always look around and see people in a worse place than we are.

As I mentioned earlier, mental illness groups are a valuable thing. I don't use a computer but I am sure there are some groups online. Maybe you could start one yourself.

It is a universal law, if we help others, we help ourselves. For those of you that hear voices, this can be very confusing. As I said, the brain is a mine field in a battlefield, so to speak. Be sure you understand humans have two tongues, one is your flesh tongue or voice and your spirit tongue which is in your mind.

All human beings are bipolar. We are all made that way. It is when you become diagnosed bipolar that your chemical balance is out of order. This can be caused by many different things. Two generations of alcoholism can cause the third generation to be bipolar. So sometimes it is a DNA thing but other times it can be a PTSD experience. It can also be caused by misuse of drugs and/or alcohol. Addiction can be a form of bipolar also. No matter what the cause, man up to it and accept that it is what it is. You or anyone else can't change it.

Let's talk a little about PTSD or post-traumatic stress disorder. I am also diagnosed with this disorder which is a result of war. I have been going to various groups for bipolar as well as PTSD. I have learned that PTSD can be caused by many different traumatic events. You may even be suffering from it along with being bipolar. This is a dual diagnosis. It can come from a rape, bad childhood or an abusive relationship. Basically, it is a stress disorder stemming from a traumatic event or events. Let's face it, life is sometimes stressful. If you are having shutdowns due to stress, you may want to talk to your doctor about it. I say again, don't be ashamed to see a psychiatrist. When I was coming up, you were looked down on if you had to see a 'shrink' but in this generation, it is not so much like that. Things are a lot more stressful now than they were and it is more acceptable to see a psychiatrist now.

In a seven-step program, I now attend, the first step is 'to seek the honor that comes from God only and no other creature'. We need not care so much what other people think. Others can think or say very hurtful things sometimes but don't let it stop you from doing what you need to do for yourself.

CHAPTER 10

Environment

Being bipolar is one of the most challenging things you will ever have to face. Try your best to get the mindset that I'll take help from anywhere I can get it.

Bipolar mania is like doing a drug or experiencing something heavenly. Once you have experienced it, you are always chasing the dragon.

That's why bipolar depression is so bad. You have experienced highs that most people haven't nor ever will. When you are depressed, it seems like hell.

Environment can make things worse. There's an old saying that says: You are known by the company you keep.

I'm not saying stay away from your friends. I'm just saying be sure you know who are your true friends.

People upset me when they say, Oh it's all in your mind. Well, it is all in your mind. But they haven't experienced the height and depth of bipolar disorder as we have. Depression with a bipolar disorder can be very dangerous. Most bipolar people commit suicide when they are in depressed state of mind. Suicide is never the answer. There are medications to help with this. It's not easy. So, accept the fact that it's a long hard journey.

Also, the manic side of bipolar can lead to suicide. But most happen on the depressed side.

Remember what I said about cycles. The chances are if you are depressed, over a period of time you will start moving up again.

I know this is a small little book, but if it helps one person it's worth it.

I still struggle with it myself. I have been battling depression for the last several months. The manic side usually doesn't last as long. You usually start losing sleep. You feel so excited you just can't sleep.

But that's when you can get into a lot of trouble.

In this summary, we have covered just about everything I have written about including environment.

So, Christ bless you on your journey in the flesh.

SUMMARY

Well, above all of the things we have talked about in this short booklet, _pray to be a teachable spirit_, no matter what faith you are. The more we learn to yield to the Holy Spirit, the further God can move us down the path of spirit. Being diagnosed with bipolar disorder is a long row to hoe. You will be dealing with it the rest of your life in the flesh. However, you can be of sound mind and be happy and healthy. You must believe this. Many things are possible to them that believe, but we must first believe it can happen. Some bipolar patients just plain give up and that is understandable. I have not met one person that hasn't given up from time to time. We talked about admitting. Even after they are diagnosed, some people reject it and keep on trying to live their lives without help. This will eventually lead to problems. You may end up in a mental hospital for a while. It's not the end of the world. In fact, it could be the dawn of you seeing that you need help. So, admitting you have a problem is only the first part. We must seek help and stick to it. Sometimes when you are clinically diagnosed bipolar, you may be able to get some financial assistance from the state. For more information, talk to your doctor or social services about this.

Purpose is something we all need. We are all here for many reasons. You may not know your ultimate purpose for being here just yet. To have the human experience is a good place to start. It is important to have the human experience, the effects of it affect us throughout eternity. It is God's will for you to be here. You may not understand that at present but keep working on improving your life. By and by, lights will start to pop on. We talked about spirituality; and again I say Jesus and His God are as much a part of my day as food and water. I couldn't write a book and not have spirituality be a part of it. I sincerely asked Jesus to come into my soul and help me when I was in Vietnam in 1972. I mostly played games with God until then. I had a relationship with Him but it was mostly an 'I want' relationship, it was not a 'Thy will be done' one. I wish all people could become true Christians. The world would abound in love if that were the case. However, not all people that call themselves Christians are true Christians, just as all people that claim to be godly are not. The spirit of love is always the 'thermometer'. We also talked about voices. There are other mental illnesses where people hear voices, but it's also not uncommon for bipolar patients. Here again, this is a grey area. There are a lot of factors that play a part in what you experience. We also talked about heart space and mind space. We talked about having two tongues or two voices, your fleshly voice and your spirit voice. The voice you use to talk to yourself in your mind is your spirit voice. God gives all human beings gifts and talents. One of these is the ability to reason, which is in a baby at a very early age and develops as you grow. The way I look at it is, all human beings are gifted with talents. You may not be aware of them at present but they develop as you grow older. The ability to communicate is a talent. Many creatures in creation have the ability to communicate. Angels both good and evil, also have the ability to communicate. We are talking about ways to communicate with angels, as I said, the human soul is a great mystery. The foundation for the word church is a drawn-out assembly of souls. It has little to do with sticks and stones. I believe the human soul is the same. It is a drawn-out assembly; you are not alone in there. So, you hear voices, that could be a good thing. I remember years ago if you told the doctors, you hear voices, the first thing was to get you in a mental institution as soon as possible. Not so frequent in this generation. People accept more now that we communicate with outside forces as well as inside forces. When I first told the psychiatrist I have now that I hear voices, she asked me 'what do the voices say to you?' She was also is a spiritual individual. I believe that is important. If you are bipolar and a spiritual person, you need to find a psychiatrist that is also. If you're not a spiritual person, that is ok too. I am learning to accept people just the way they are. My heart still goes out to you. We talked about circles and cycles. Study your bipolar disorder, there probably are cycles involved. If this is the case, knowing about them could help with the highs and lows not going too far. It is a lot about balance. We are seeking a middle ground so to speak. All human beings have highs and lows, it's just that when you are diagnosed bipolar, you need a little extra help with the chemical imbalance. We also talked about the very present or 'Isma' dimension. Our minds can wander off into the past and the future, but it is in the very present where all change takes place. Try and focus on the present as much as possible. We have talked about a lot of things in this little book. Some things you had probably heard of and some you may not. We must agree to disagree about some things. I hope it has helped you better understand bipolar disorder, in yourself or maybe someone you know. Again, this book is strictly from a patient's point of view. Above all things that I have written, I wish you wellness!